DIABETIC RENAL DIET COOKBOOK

Flavorful Recipes for Managing Diabetes & Kidney Disease

T. John

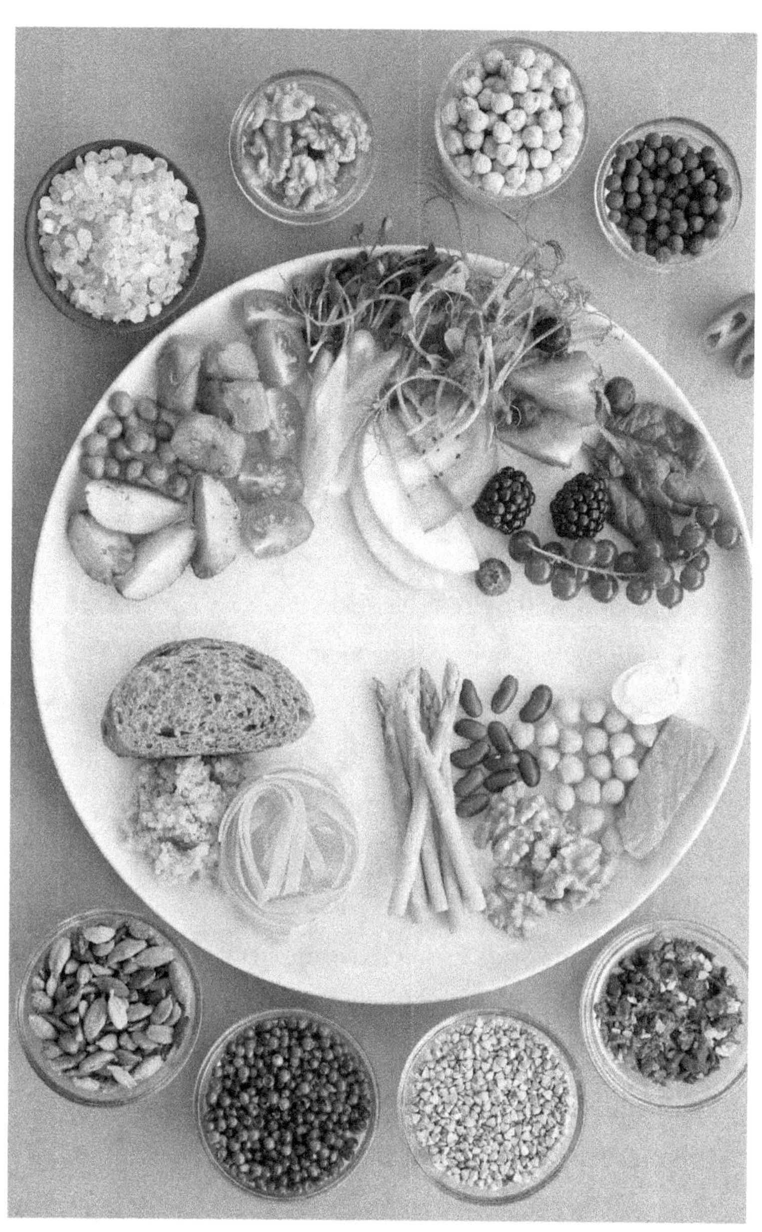

TABLE OF CONTENTS

Chapter 5: Snacks and Appetizers 89

INTRODUCTION

I magine your body as a delicate ecosystem, where your kidneys act as the tireless filtration system, ensuring the balance of vital fluids and minerals. Now, introduce diabetes, a mischievous intruder that throws this ecosystem into disarray, potentially targeting even your kidneys. This is where the diabetic renal diet steps in, not as a restrictive prison, but as a transformative tool to restore harmony and safeguard your renal health.

The Delicate Dance Between Diabetes and Kidneys:

Diabetes, with its elevated blood sugar levels, can damage blood vessels throughout the body, including those nourishing your kidneys. This damage can lead to a condition called diabetic nephropathy, where your kidneys struggle to filter waste effectively. Over time, this can progress to chronic kidney disease, a serious complication.

The Power of Food as Medicine:

But here's the good news: you're not at the mercy of this progression. The diabetic renal diet, crafted in collaboration with your healthcare team, becomes your personal chef, whipping up dishes that nourish both your body and your kidneys. It's not just about "what" you eat, but "how" you orchestrate your meals to create a symphony of wellness.

The Harmony of Macronutrients:

- **Carbohydrates**: The delicate melody of carbs. Choose complex carbohydrates like whole grains, fruits, and vegetables, which release glucose slowly, preventing blood sugar spikes. Avoid refined carbs like white bread and sugary drinks, the villainous crescendos that disrupt your renal harmony.

- **Protein**: The steady bassline of protein. While crucial for building and repairing tissues, excessive protein can strain your kidneys. Aim for moderate amounts, prioritizing plant-based sources like beans and lentils, while limiting animal proteins.

- **Fats**: The rhythmic pulse of fats. Opt for healthy fats like olive oil, avocados, and fatty fish, rich in omega-3s, which can help lower blood pressure and protect your kidneys. Avoid saturated and trans fats, the discordant notes that contribute to inflammation and kidney damage.

The Orchestration of Nutrients:

Beyond the macronutrients, a diabetic renal diet focuses on the finer notes:

- **Sodium**: The quiet enemy lurking in processed foods. Limit sodium intake to reduce fluid buildup and protect your blood pressure, a key factor in renal health.

- **Potassium**: The essential counterpart to sodium. Maintain proper potassium levels, but be mindful, as excessive potassium can also be harmful. Your doctor can guide you on the right balance.

- **Phosphorus**: The silent threat. Phosphorus, found in processed meats and dairy products, can build up in the kidneys and contribute to bone disease. Choose low-phosphorus options or limit your intake.

The Symphony of Deliciousness:

Remember, a diabetic renal diet is not a bland, monotonous dirge. It's a vibrant orchestra of flavor, where spices, herbs, and creative culinary combinations replace salt as the conductor. Explore new ingredients, experiment with textures, and discover the joy of cooking kidney-friendly dishes that tantalize your taste buds.

The Final Note:

The journey of managing diabetes and protecting your renal health is a continuous performance, not a one-time act. Embrace the diabetic renal diet as your guide, learn its intricacies, and adapt it to your unique preferences. With each bite, you become the maestro of your own wellness, composing a symphony of health that resonates throughout your body and protects your precious kidneys.

Remember, this is just a starting point. Your healthcare team, including your doctor and registered dietitian, are your invaluable collaborators in this journey. They can personalize the diabetic renal diet to your specific needs and provide ongoing support as you navigate this delicate dance between food and health. So, take a deep breath, trust the rhythm of your body, and embark on this transformative journey towards a healthier, kidney-harmonious you.

Chapter 1: 30-Day Meal Plan

Week 1:

Day 1:

- Breakfast: Quinoa and Berry Breakfast Bowl
- Lunch: Grilled Chicken Salad with Balsamic Vinaigrette
- Dinner: Baked Lemon Herb Chicken
- Snack: Guacamole with Veggie Sticks
- Dessert: Sugar-Free Berry Sorbet

Day 2:

- Breakfast: Veggie Omelette with Spinach and Feta
- Lunch: Lentil Soup with Vegetables
- Dinner: Cauliflower Fried Rice with Shrimp
- Snack: Greek Yogurt and Cucumber Dip
- Dessert: Dark Chocolate and Almond Clusters

Day 3:

- Breakfast: Chia Seed Pudding with Almond Milk
- Lunch: Quinoa and Black Bean Bowl

- Dinner: Grilled Salmon with Dill Sauce
- Snack: Hummus with Carrot and Celery Sticks
- Dessert: Coconut and Chia Seed Pudding

Day 4:

- Breakfast: Whole Grain Pancakes with Sugar-Free Syrup
- Lunch: Shrimp and Avocado Lettuce Wraps
- Dinner: Vegetarian Zoodle Stir-Fry
- Snack: Deviled Eggs with Avocado
- Dessert: Baked Apple with Cinnamon

Day 5:

- Breakfast: Greek Yogurt Parfait with Fresh Berries
- Lunch: Turkey and Vegetable Stir-Fry
- Dinner: Stuffed Bell Peppers with Ground Turkey
- Snack: Spicy Edamame
- Dessert: Greek Yogurt Cheesecake Bites

Day 6:

- Breakfast: Avocado and Tomato Breakfast Wrap
- Lunch: Chickpea and Vegetable Curry

- Dinner: Roasted Garlic and Rosemary Pork Tenderloin
- Snack: Cottage Cheese and Pineapple Skewers
- Dessert: Avocado Chocolate Mousse

Day 7:

- Breakfast: Sweet Potato Hash with Poached Eggs
- Lunch: Spinach and Feta Stuffed Chicken Breast
- Dinner: Eggplant Parmesan with Whole Wheat Pasta
- Snack: Roasted Red Pepper and Feta Dip
- Dessert: Pumpkin Pie Chia Pudding

Week 2:

Day 8:

- Breakfast: Nutty Granola with Low-Glycemic Fruits
- Lunch: Tuna Salad Lettuce Wraps
- Dinner: Cilantro Lime Grilled Chicken
- Snack: Almond and Pumpkin Seed Trail Mix
- Dessert: Berry and Almond Tart

Day 9:

- Breakfast: Spinach and Mushroom Breakfast Casserole
- Lunch: Cauliflower and Broccoli Gratin
- Dinner: Quinoa and Vegetable Stuffed Peppers
- Snack: Caprese Skewers with Balsamic Glaze
- Dessert: Lemon Blueberry Parfait

Day 10:

- Breakfast: Salmon and Cream Cheese Bagel Thin
- Lunch: Caprese Salad with Balsamic Glaze
- Dinner: Blackened Tilapia with Mango Salsa
- Snack: Smoked Salmon Cucumber Bites
- Dessert: Pistachio and Cranberry Energy Bites

Day 11:

- Breakfast: Oatmeal with Sliced Almonds and Berries
- Lunch: Eggplant and Zucchini Lasagna
- Dinner: Spaghetti Squash with Tomato Basil Sauce
- Snack: Kale Chips with Sea Salt
- Dessert: Cinnamon Baked Pears

Day 12:

- Breakfast: Protein-Packed Breakfast Burrito
- Lunch: Mediterranean Hummus Wrap
- Dinner: Chicken and Vegetable Skewers
- Snack: Baked Sweet Potato Fries
- Dessert: Almond Flour Banana Bread

Day 13:

- Breakfast: Cottage Cheese and Pineapple Bowl
- Lunch: Salmon and Quinoa Patties
- Dinner: Creamy Mushroom and Spinach Risotto
- Snack: Avocado and Black Bean Salsa
- Dessert: Raspberry and Coconut Chia Jam

Day 14:

- Breakfast: Turkey Sausage and Vegetable Scramble
- Lunch: Turkey and Sweet Potato Chili
- Dinner: Baked Cod with Lemon and Herbs
- Snack: Zucchini and Parmesan Crisps
- Dessert: Vanilla Bean Panna Cotta

Week 3:

Day 15:

- Breakfast: Banana Walnut Muffins (Sugar-Free)
- Lunch: Roasted Vegetable Quiche
- Dinner: Teriyaki Tofu Stir-Fry
- Snack: Mixed Berry Smoothie Bowl
- Dessert: Mint Chocolate Avocado Popsicles

Day 16:

- Breakfast: Quinoa and Berry Breakfast Bowl
- Lunch: Grilled Chicken Salad with Balsamic Vinaigrette
- Dinner: Baked Lemon Herb Chicken
- Snack: Guacamole with Veggie Sticks
- Dessert: Sugar-Free Berry Sorbet

Day 17:

- Breakfast: Veggie Omelette with Spinach and Feta
- Lunch: Lentil Soup with Vegetables
- Dinner: Cauliflower Fried Rice with Shrimp
- Snack: Greek Yogurt and Cucumber Dip
- Dessert: Dark Chocolate and Almond Clusters

Day 18:

- Breakfast: Chia Seed Pudding with Almond Milk
- Lunch: Quinoa and Black Bean Bowl
- Dinner: Grilled Salmon with Dill Sauce
- Snack: Hummus with Carrot and Celery Sticks
- Dessert: Coconut and Chia Seed Pudding

Day 19:

- Breakfast: Whole Grain Pancakes with Sugar-Free Syrup
- Lunch: Shrimp and Avocado Lettuce Wraps
- Dinner: Vegetarian Zoodle Stir-Fry
- Snack: Deviled Eggs with Avocado
- Dessert: Baked Apple with Cinnamon

Day 20:

- Breakfast: Greek Yogurt Parfait with Fresh Berries
- Lunch: Turkey and Vegetable Stir-Fry
- Dinner: Stuffed Bell Peppers with Ground Turkey
- Snack: Spicy Edamame
- Dessert: Greek Yogurt Cheesecake Bites

Day 21:

- Breakfast: Avocado and Tomato Breakfast Wrap
- Lunch: Chickpea and Vegetable Curry
- Dinner: Roasted Garlic and Rosemary Pork Tenderloin
- Snack: Cottage Cheese and Pineapple Skewers
- Dessert: Avocado Chocolate Mousse

Week 4:

Day 22:

- Breakfast: Sweet Potato Hash with Poached Eggs
- Lunch: Spinach and Feta Stuffed Chicken Breast
- Dinner: Eggplant Parmesan with Whole Wheat Pasta
- Snack: Roasted Red Pepper and Feta Dip
- Dessert: Pumpkin Pie Chia Pudding

Day 23:

- Breakfast: Nutty Granola with Low-Glycemic Fruits
- Lunch: Tuna Salad Lettuce Wraps
- Dinner: Cilantro Lime Grilled Chicken
- Snack: Almond and Pumpkin Seed Trail Mix
- Dessert: Berry and Almond Tart

Day 24:

- Breakfast: Spinach and Mushroom Breakfast Casserole
- Lunch: Cauliflower and Broccoli Gratin
- Dinner: Quinoa and Vegetable Stuffed Peppers
- Snack: Caprese Skewers with Balsamic Glaze
- Dessert: Lemon Blueberry Parfait

Day 25:

- Breakfast: Salmon and Cream Cheese Bagel Thin
- Lunch: Caprese Salad with Balsamic Glaze
- Dinner: Blackened Tilapia with Mango Salsa
- Snack: Smoked Salmon Cucumber Bites
- Dessert: Pistachio and Cranberry Energy Bites

Day 26:

- Breakfast: Oatmeal with Sliced Almonds and Berries
- Lunch: Eggplant and Zucchini Lasagna
- Dinner: Spaghetti Squash with Tomato Basil Sauce
- Snack: Kale Chips with Sea Salt
- Dessert: Cinnamon Baked Pears

Day 27:

- Breakfast: Protein-Packed Breakfast Burrito
- Lunch: Mediterranean Hummus Wrap
- Dinner: Chicken and Vegetable Skewers
- Snack: Baked Sweet Potato Fries
- Dessert: Almond Flour Banana Bread

Day 28:

- Breakfast: Cottage Cheese and Pineapple Bowl
- Lunch: Salmon and Quinoa Patties
- Dinner: Creamy Mushroom and Spinach Risotto
- Snack: Avocado and Black Bean Salsa
- Dessert: Raspberry and Coconut Chia Jam

Day 29:

- Breakfast: Turkey Sausage and Vegetable Scramble
- Lunch: Turkey and Sweet Potato Chili
- Dinner: Baked Cod with Lemon and Herbs
- Snack: Zucchini and Parmesan Crisps
- Dessert: Vanilla Bean Panna Cotta

Day 30:

- Breakfast: Banana Walnut Muffins (Sugar-Free)
- Lunch: Roasted Vegetable Quiche
- Dinner: Teriyaki Tofu Stir-Fry
- Snack: Mixed Berry Smoothie Bowl
- Dessert: Mint Chocolate Avocado Popsicles

Chapter 2: Breakfast Recipes

These recipes are not just nourishing but also bursting with flavors that will make your mornings a joy. Each dish is crafted with precision to ensure a balance of essential nutrients while keeping the taste buds satisfied.

Quinoa and Berry Breakfast Bowl

Ingredients:

- 1/2 cup quinoa
- 1 cup mixed berries (strawberries, blueberries, raspberries)
- 1 tablespoon honey
- 1/4 cup chopped almonds
- 1/2 teaspoon vanilla extract

Instructions:

1. Rinse quinoa thoroughly and cook according to package instructions.
2. In a bowl, combine cooked quinoa, mixed berries, honey, chopped almonds, and vanilla extract.

3. Mix well and enjoy!

Nutrition Information (per serving):

- Calories: 250

- Protein: 8g

- Carbohydrates: 40g

- Fat: 7g

- Sodium: 10mg

- Potassium: 320mg

- Phosphorus: 120mg

- Portion Size: 1 bowl

Veggie Omelette with Spinach and Feta

Ingredients:

- 2 eggs
- 1/4 cup spinach, chopped
- 2 tablespoons feta cheese, crumbled
- 1/4 cup bell peppers, diced
- Salt and pepper to taste

Instructions:

1. Whisk eggs in a bowl and season with salt and pepper.
2. Heat a non-stick pan and pour in the whisked eggs.
3. Add spinach, feta cheese, and bell peppers on one side of the omelette.
4. Fold the omelette in half and cook until eggs are fully set.

Nutrition Information (per serving):

- Calories: 180
- Protein: 14g
- Carbohydrates: 4g
- Fat: 12g
- Sodium: 250mg
- Potassium: 200mg
- Phosphorus: 150mg
- Portion Size: 1 omelette

Chia Seed Pudding with Almond Milk

Ingredients:

- 3 tablespoons chia seeds

- 1 cup unsweetened almond milk
- 1/2 teaspoon vanilla extract
- 1 tablespoon maple syrup (optional)
- Fresh berries for topping

Instructions:

1. In a bowl, mix chia seeds, almond milk, vanilla extract, and maple syrup (if using).
2. Stir well, ensuring chia seeds are evenly distributed.
3. Refrigerate for at least 4 hours or overnight.
4. Top with fresh berries before serving.

Nutrition Information (per serving):

- Calories: 150
- Protein: 5g
- Carbohydrates: 15g
- Fat: 9g
- Sodium: 80mg
- Potassium: 120mg
- Phosphorus: 100mg
- Portion Size: 1 pudding cup

Whole Grain Pancakes with Sugar-Free Syrup

Ingredients:

- 1/2 cup whole wheat flour
- 1/2 cup oat flour
- 1 teaspoon baking powder
- 1/2 teaspoon cinnamon
- 1/2 cup milk (dairy or plant-based)
- 1 egg
- Sugar-free syrup for topping

Instructions:

1. In a bowl, mix whole wheat flour, oat flour, baking powder, and cinnamon.
2. Add milk and egg, stirring until just combined.
3. Pour batter onto a hot, greased griddle and cook until bubbles form.
4. Flip and cook until golden brown. Serve with sugar-free syrup.

Nutrition Information (per serving):

- Calories: 220

- Protein: 9g

- Carbohydrates: 30g

- Fat: 7g

- Sodium: 180mg

- Potassium: 160mg

- Phosphorus: 120mg

- Portion Size: 2 pancakes

Greek Yogurt Parfait with Fresh Berries

Ingredients:

- 1 cup Greek yogurt
- 1/2 cup granola (low-phosphorus)
- 1/2 cup fresh mixed berries
- 1 tablespoon honey

Instructions:

1. In a glass or bowl, layer Greek yogurt, granola, and fresh berries.
2. Drizzle honey on top for added sweetness.
3. Repeat the layers until the container is filled.

4. Enjoy the delightful combination of textures and flavors.

Nutrition Information (per serving):

- Calories: 280
- Protein: 15g
- Carbohydrates: 35g
- Fat: 8g
- Sodium: 60mg
- Potassium: 200mg
- Phosphorus: 150mg
- Portion Size: 1 parfait

Avocado and Tomato Breakfast Wrap

Ingredients:

- 1 whole-grain tortilla
- 1/2 avocado, sliced
- 1 medium tomato, diced
- 2 eggs, scrambled
- Salt and pepper to taste

Instructions:

1. Warm the tortilla in a dry pan or microwave.

2. Spread avocado slices on the tortilla.

3. In the same pan, scramble the eggs and season with salt and pepper.

4. Place the scrambled eggs and diced tomatoes on the tortilla, then fold and serve.

Nutrition Information (per serving):

- Calories: 320
- Protein: 14g
- Carbohydrates: 28g
- Fat: 18g
- Sodium: 200mg
- Potassium: 400mg
- Phosphorus: 200mg
- Portion Size: 1 wrap

Sweet Potato Hash with Poached Eggs

Ingredients:

- 1 medium sweet potato, grated
- 1/2 onion, diced
- 2 eggs, poached
- 1 tablespoon olive oil
- Salt and pepper to taste

Instructions:

1. In a skillet, sauté grated sweet potato and diced onion in olive oil until tender.
2. Season with salt and pepper.
3. Poach eggs in simmering water until whites are set but yolks remain runny.
4. Serve the sweet potato hash topped with poached eggs.

Nutrition Information (per serving):

- Calories: 280
- Protein: 12g
- Carbohydrates: 30g
- Fat: 14g
- Sodium: 120mg
- Potassium: 450mg

- Phosphorus: 150mg
- Portion Size: 1 serving

Nutty Granola with Low-Glycemic Fruits

Ingredients:

- 1 cup low-phosphorus granola
- 1/4 cup almonds, chopped
- 1/4 cup walnuts, chopped
- 1/2 cup mixed low-glycemic fruits (e.g., berries, cherries)
- 1 cup unsweetened almond milk

Instructions:

1. Combine granola, chopped almonds, and walnuts in a bowl.
2. Add mixed low-glycemic fruits on top.
3. Pour almond milk over the mixture.
4. Stir gently and savor the crunchy goodness.

Nutrition Information (per serving):

- Calories: 320

- Protein: 8g

- Carbohydrates: 40g

- Fat: 16g

- Sodium: 80mg

- Potassium: 180mg

- Phosphorus: 120mg

- Portion Size: 1 bowl

Spinach and Mushroom Breakfast Casserole

Ingredients:

- 2 cups spinach, chopped

- 1 cup mushrooms, sliced

- 1/2 cup feta cheese, crumbled

- 6 eggs, beaten

- 1 cup milk (dairy or plant-based)

- Salt and pepper to taste

Instructions:

1. Preheat the oven to 350°F (175°C).
2. In a greased baking dish, layer spinach, mushrooms, and feta cheese.
3. In a bowl, whisk together eggs, milk, salt, and pepper.
4. Pour the egg mixture over the veggies and cheese.
5. Bake for 25-30 minutes or until the center is set.

Nutrition Information (per serving):

- Calories: 230
- Protein: 15g
- Carbohydrates: 6g
- Fat: 16g
- Sodium: 320mg
- Potassium: 300mg
- Phosphorus: 200mg
- Portion Size: 1 slice

Salmon and Cream Cheese Bagel Thin

Ingredients:

- 1 whole-grain bagel thin

- 2 ounces smoked salmon

- 2 tablespoons cream cheese (low-fat)

- 1 tablespoon capers

- Fresh dill for garnish

Instructions:

1. Toast the bagel thin to your liking.

2. Spread cream cheese on each half of the bagel.

3. Layer smoked salmon on top and sprinkle with capers.

4. Garnish with fresh dill and enjoy this delightful open-faced sandwich.

Nutrition Information (per serving):

- Calories: 280

- Protein: 18g

- Carbohydrates: 30g

- Fat: 10g

- Sodium: 480mg

- Potassium: 200mg

- Phosphorus: 180mg

- Portion Size: 1 bagel thin

Oatmeal with Sliced Almonds and Berries

Ingredients:

- 1/2 cup rolled oats

- 1 cup water or milk (dairy or plant-based)

- 1/4 cup sliced almonds

- 1/2 cup mixed berries (strawberries, blueberries)

Instructions:

1. Cook rolled oats in water or milk according to package instructions.

2. Once cooked, top with sliced almonds and mixed berries.

3. Stir gently and let the berries release their natural sweetness.

4. Enjoy a warm and hearty bowl of oatmeal.

Nutrition Information (per serving):

- Calories: 270
- Protein: 10g
- Carbohydrates: 35g
- Fat: 10g
- Sodium: 20mg
- Potassium: 230mg
- Phosphorus: 180mg
- Portion Size: 1 bowl

Protein-Packed Breakfast Burrito

Ingredients:

- 1 whole-grain tortilla
- 1/2 cup black beans, drained and rinsed
- 2 eggs, scrambled
- 1/4 cup salsa
- 1/4 cup shredded low-fat cheese

Instructions:

1. Warm the tortilla in a dry pan or microwave.
2. Layer black beans, scrambled eggs, salsa, and shredded cheese on the tortilla.

3. Fold into a burrito and enjoy this protein-packed breakfast.

Nutrition Information (per serving):

- Calories: 300
- Protein: 20g
- Carbohydrates: 30g
- Fat: 10g
- Sodium: 520mg
- Potassium: 280mg
- Phosphorus: 200mg
- Portion Size: 1 burrito

Cottage Cheese and Pineapple Bowl

Ingredients:

- 1 cup low-fat cottage cheese
- 1/2 cup fresh pineapple chunks
- 1 tablespoon honey
- 1 tablespoon chopped mint (optional)

Instructions:

1. In a bowl, combine cottage cheese and fresh pineapple chunks.

2. Drizzle with honey and sprinkle chopped mint for added freshness.

3. Mix gently and savor the sweet and savory combination.

Nutrition Information (per serving):

- Calories: 220
- Protein: 20g
- Carbohydrates: 25g
- Fat: 4g
- Sodium: 320mg
- Potassium: 280mg
- Phosphorus: 180mg
- Portion Size: 1 bowl

Turkey Sausage and Vegetable Scramble

Ingredients:

- 2 turkey sausage links, sliced
- 1/2 bell pepper, diced
- 1/2 zucchini, diced
- 2 eggs, beaten
- Salt and pepper to taste

Instructions:

1. In a skillet, cook turkey sausage slices until browned.
2. Add diced bell pepper and zucchini, sauté until tender.
3. Pour beaten eggs over the mixture, season with salt and pepper.
4. Scramble until eggs are cooked through. Serve warm.

Nutrition Information (per serving):

- Calories: 250
- Protein: 18g
- Carbohydrates: 8g
- Fat: 15g
- Sodium: 480mg
- Potassium: 300mg

- Phosphorus: 200mg

- Portion Size: 1 serving

Banana Walnut Muffins (Sugar-Free)

Ingredients:

- 2 ripe bananas, mashed

- 1/2 cup chopped walnuts

- 2 cups almond flour

- 3 eggs

- 1 teaspoon baking powder

- 1/2 teaspoon cinnamon

Instructions:

1. Preheat the oven to 350°F (175°C) and line a muffin tin with paper liners.

2. In a bowl, mix mashed bananas, chopped walnuts, almond flour, eggs, baking powder, and cinnamon.

3. Spoon the batter into muffin cups and bake for 20-25 minutes or until a toothpick comes out clean.

Nutrition Information (per muffin):

- Calories: 180
- Protein: 7g
- Carbohydrates: 12g
- Fat: 13g
- Sodium: 30mg
- Potassium: 200mg
- Phosphorus: 100mg
- Portion Size: 1 muffin

These nutrient-rich and flavorful dishes not only bring a burst of taste to your midday meal but also adhere to the dietary guidelines essential for managing your health effectively.

Grilled Chicken Salad with Balsamic Vinaigrette

Ingredients:

- 1 boneless, skinless chicken breast
- 2 cups mixed salad greens
- 1 cup cherry tomatoes, halved
- 1/4 cup cucumber, sliced
- 2 tablespoons feta cheese, crumbled
- 2 tablespoons balsamic vinaigrette dressing

Instructions:

1. Season the chicken breast with salt and pepper.
2. Grill the chicken until fully cooked.
3. Slice the grilled chicken into strips.

4. In a large bowl, combine salad greens, cherry tomatoes, cucumber, and grilled chicken.

5. Sprinkle feta cheese on top.

6. Drizzle balsamic vinaigrette dressing over the salad.

7. Toss gently and serve.

Nutrition Information:

- Calories: 350

- Protein: 30g

- Carbohydrates: 15g

- Fat: 18g

- Sodium: 400mg

- Potassium: 550mg

- Phosphorus: 200mg

- Portion Size: 1 serving

Lentil Soup with Vegetables

Ingredients:

- 1 cup dry lentils, rinsed

- 4 cups vegetable broth

- 1 onion, diced

- 2 carrots, chopped

- 2 celery stalks, chopped
- 2 cloves garlic, minced
- 1 teaspoon cumin
- 1/2 teaspoon smoked paprika
- Salt and pepper to taste

Instructions:

1. In a large pot, combine lentils, vegetable broth, onion, carrots, celery, garlic, cumin, smoked paprika, salt, and pepper.
2. Bring to a boil, then reduce heat and simmer until lentils are tender.
3. Adjust seasoning to taste.
4. Serve hot.

Nutrition Information:

- Calories: 280
- Protein: 18g
- Carbohydrates: 45g
- Fat: 2g
- Sodium: 600mg
- Potassium: 700mg

- Phosphorus: 180mg

- Portion Size: 1 cup

Quinoa and Black Bean Bowl

Ingredients:

- 1 cup cooked quinoa

- 1 cup black beans, drained and rinsed

- 1 cup corn kernels (fresh or frozen)

- 1 red bell pepper, diced

- 1/4 cup fresh cilantro, chopped

- 1 tablespoon olive oil

- Juice of 1 lime

- Salt and pepper to taste

Instructions:

1. In a large bowl, combine cooked quinoa, black beans, corn, red bell pepper, and cilantro.

2. Drizzle olive oil and lime juice over the mixture.

3. Season with salt and pepper.

4. Toss gently until well combined.

5. Serve at room temperature.

Nutrition Information:

- Calories: 320
- Protein: 15g
- Carbohydrates: 50g
- Fat: 8g
- Sodium: 300mg
- Potassium: 450mg
- Phosphorus: 200mg
- Portion Size: 1 serving

Shrimp and Avocado Lettuce Wraps

Ingredients:

- 1/2 pound shrimp, peeled and deveined
- 1 avocado, diced
- 1 cup cherry tomatoes, halved
- 1/4 cup red onion, finely chopped
- 2 tablespoons cilantro, chopped
- 1 tablespoon olive oil
- Juice of 1 lemon
- Salt and pepper to taste
- Butter lettuce leaves for wrapping

Instructions:

1. Cook shrimp in olive oil until pink and opaque.
2. In a bowl, combine shrimp, avocado, cherry tomatoes, red onion, cilantro, olive oil, lemon juice, salt, and pepper.
3. Spoon the mixture into butter lettuce leaves.
4. Serve as wraps.

Nutrition Information:

- Calories: 280
- Protein: 20g
- Carbohydrates: 15g
- Fat: 15g
- Sodium: 250mg
- Potassium: 400mg
- Phosphorus: 180mg
- Portion Size: 2 wraps

Turkey and Vegetable Stir-Fry

Ingredients:

- 1/2 pound lean ground turkey

- 2 cups mixed stir-fry vegetables (broccoli, bell peppers, snap peas)
- 1 tablespoon low-sodium soy sauce
- 1 tablespoon hoisin sauce
- 1 teaspoon sesame oil
- 1 teaspoon ginger, minced
- 2 cloves garlic, minced
- 2 green onions, sliced

Instructions:

1. In a wok or skillet, brown ground turkey until fully cooked.
2. Add stir-fry vegetables and stir-fry for 3-5 minutes.
3. In a small bowl, mix soy sauce, hoisin sauce, sesame oil, ginger, and garlic.
4. Pour the sauce over the turkey and vegetables, stirring to combine.
5. Cook for an additional 2-3 minutes.
6. Garnish with sliced green onions.

Nutrition Information:

- Calories: 280

- Protein: 25g

- Carbohydrates: 15g

- Fat: 12g

- Sodium: 450mg

- Potassium: 380mg

- Phosphorus: 200mg

- Portion Size: 1 serving

Chickpea and Vegetable Curry

Ingredients:

- 1 can (15 oz) chickpeas, drained and rinsed

- 1 cup cauliflower florets

- 1 cup sweet potatoes, diced

- 1 cup spinach leaves

- 1 can (14 oz) diced tomatoes

- 1 onion, finely chopped

- 2 cloves garlic, minced

- 1 tablespoon curry powder

- 1 teaspoon cumin

- 1 teaspoon turmeric

- Salt and pepper to taste

Instructions:

1. In a large pot, sauté onions and garlic until softened.

2. Add curry powder, cumin, turmeric, salt, and pepper; stir well.

3. Add chickpeas, cauliflower, sweet potatoes, diced tomatoes, and enough water to cover.

4. Simmer until vegetables are tender.

5. Stir in spinach just before serving.

Nutrition Information:

- Calories: 320
- Protein: 15g
- Carbohydrates: 55g
- Fat: 5g
- Sodium: 500mg
- Potassium: 600mg
- Phosphorus: 180mg
- Portion Size: 1 serving

Spinach and Feta Stuffed Chicken Breast

Ingredients:

- 2 boneless, skinless chicken breasts
- 2 cups fresh spinach, chopped
- 1/4 cup feta cheese, crumbled
- 2 tablespoons olive oil
- 1 teaspoon garlic powder
- 1 teaspoon dried oregano
- Salt and pepper to taste

Instructions:

1. Preheat the oven to 375°F (190°C).
2. In a skillet, sauté spinach in olive oil until wilted.
3. Butterfly the chicken breasts and season with garlic powder, oregano, salt, and pepper.
4. Stuff each chicken breast with sautéed spinach and feta cheese.
5. Secure with toothpicks and bake for 25-30 minutes or until chicken is cooked through.
6. Remove toothpicks before serving.

Nutrition Information:

- Calories: 320
- Protein: 35g
- Carbohydrates: 4g
- Fat: 18g
- Sodium: 400mg
- Potassium: 500mg
- Phosphorus: 250mg
- Portion Size: 1 serving

Tuna Salad Lettuce Wraps

Ingredients:

- 2 cans (5 oz each) tuna in water, drained
- 1/4 cup celery, finely chopped
- 1/4 cup red onion, finely chopped
- 2 tablespoons mayonnaise (low-fat)
- 1 tablespoon Dijon mustard
- 1 teaspoon lemon juice
- Salt and pepper to taste
- Butter lettuce leaves for wrapping

Instructions:

1. In a bowl, combine tuna, celery, red onion, mayonnaise, Dijon mustard, lemon juice, salt, and pepper.
2. Mix until well combined.
3. Spoon the tuna salad into butter lettuce leaves.
4. Serve as wraps.

Nutrition Information:

- Calories: 250
- Protein: 25g
- Carbohydrates: 5g
- Fat: 15g
- Sodium: 400mg
- Potassium: 300mg
- Phosphorus: 180mg
- Portion Size: 2 wraps

Cauliflower and Broccoli Gratin

Ingredients:

- 2 cups cauliflower florets
- 2 cups broccoli florets

- 1 cup shredded cheddar cheese
- 1/2 cup grated Parmesan cheese
- 1 cup low-fat milk
- 2 tablespoons whole wheat flour
- 2 tablespoons unsalted butter
- 1 teaspoon Dijon mustard
- 1/2 teaspoon nutmeg
- Salt and pepper to taste

Instructions:

1. Steam cauliflower and broccoli until tender. Place in a baking dish.
2. In a saucepan, melt butter and whisk in flour to create a roux.
3. Gradually add milk, stirring continuously until the mixture thickens.
4. Stir in Dijon mustard, nutmeg, salt, and pepper.
5. Pour the sauce over the vegetables in the baking dish.
6. Top with shredded cheddar and Parmesan cheese.
7. Bake in the oven at 350°F (180°C) until the cheese is melted and golden.

Nutrition Information:

- Calories: 280
- Protein: 15g
- Carbohydrates: 20g
- Fat: 16g
- Sodium: 400mg
- Potassium: 450mg
- Phosphorus: 200mg
- Portion Size: 1 serving

Caprese Salad with Balsamic Glaze

Ingredients:

- 2 large tomatoes, sliced
- 1 cup fresh mozzarella, sliced
- 1/4 cup fresh basil leaves
- 2 tablespoons balsamic glaze
- 1 tablespoon extra virgin olive oil
- Salt and pepper to taste

Instructions:

1. Arrange alternating slices of tomatoes and mozzarella on a serving platter.

2. Tuck fresh basil leaves between the slices.

3. Drizzle with balsamic glaze and olive oil.

4. Sprinkle with salt and pepper.

5. Serve chilled.

Nutrition Information:

- Calories: 250

- Protein: 15g

- Carbohydrates: 10g

- Fat: 18g

- Sodium: 300mg

- Potassium: 400mg

- Phosphorus: 180mg

- Portion Size: 1 serving

Eggplant and Zucchini Lasagna

Ingredients:

- 1 large eggplant, thinly sliced

- 2 medium zucchinis, thinly sliced

- 2 cups low-sodium marinara sauce

- 1 cup part-skim ricotta cheese

- 1 cup shredded mozzarella cheese

- 1/4 cup grated Parmesan cheese
- 2 cloves garlic, minced
- 1 teaspoon dried oregano
- Salt and pepper to taste

Instructions:

1. Preheat the oven to 375°F (190°C).
2. In a bowl, combine ricotta cheese, minced garlic, dried oregano, salt, and pepper.
3. In a baking dish, layer eggplant, zucchini, marinara sauce, ricotta mixture, and mozzarella cheese.
4. Repeat the layers, finishing with a layer of mozzarella on top.
5. Sprinkle Parmesan cheese over the top layer.
6. Bake for 35-40 minutes or until the vegetables are tender and the cheese is bubbly.

Nutrition Information:

- Calories: 320
- Protein: 20g
- Carbohydrates: 25g
- Fat: 15g

- Sodium: 500mg

- Potassium: 600mg

- Phosphorus: 200mg

- Portion Size: 1 serving

Mediterranean Hummus Wrap

Ingredients:

- 1 whole wheat wrap

- 1/2 cup hummus

- 1/2 cup cucumber, sliced

- 1/2 cup cherry tomatoes, halved

- 1/4 cup Kalamata olives, sliced

- 1/4 cup feta cheese, crumbled

- Fresh parsley for garnish

Instructions:

1. Spread hummus over the whole wheat wrap.

2. Layer with cucumber, cherry tomatoes, Kalamata olives, and feta cheese.

3. Garnish with fresh parsley.

4. Roll up the wrap and slice in half.

Nutrition Information:

- Calories: 300
- Protein: 12g
- Carbohydrates: 30g
- Fat: 15g
- Sodium: 550mg
- Potassium: 400mg
- Phosphorus: 180mg
- Portion Size: 1 serving

Salmon and Quinoa Patties

Ingredients:

- 1 can (14 oz) pink salmon, drained and flaked
- 1 cup cooked quinoa
- 1/4 cup whole wheat breadcrumbs
- 1/4 cup green onions, finely chopped
- 1 egg, beaten
- 1 tablespoon Dijon mustard
- 1 teaspoon lemon zest
- 1/2 teaspoon dried dill
- Salt and pepper to taste
- 2 tablespoons olive oil for cooking

Instructions:

1. In a bowl, combine salmon, cooked quinoa, breadcrumbs, green onions, egg, Dijon mustard, lemon zest, dried dill, salt, and pepper.
2. Form the mixture into patties.
3. Heat olive oil in a skillet over medium heat.
4. Cook the patties until golden brown on each side.
5. Serve hot.

Nutrition Information:

- Calories: 280
- Protein: 20g
- Carbohydrates: 20g
- Fat: 12g
- Sodium: 450mg
- Potassium: 500mg
- Phosphorus: 200mg
- Portion Size: 2 patties

Turkey and Sweet Potato Chili

Ingredients:

- 1 pound ground turkey

- 1 large sweet potato, peeled and diced

- 1 can (14 oz) diced tomatoes

- 1 can (15 oz) black beans, drained and rinsed

- 1 cup low-sodium chicken broth

- 1 onion, diced

- 2 cloves garlic, minced

- 2 tablespoons chili powder

- 1 teaspoon cumin

- 1 teaspoon paprika

- Salt and pepper to taste

Instructions:

1. In a large pot, brown ground turkey with onion and garlic.

2. Add sweet potato, diced tomatoes, black beans, chicken broth, chili powder, cumin, paprika, salt, and pepper.

3. Simmer until sweet potatoes are tender and flavors are well combined.

4. Adjust seasoning if needed.

5. Serve hot.

Nutrition Information:

- Calories: 300
- Protein: 25g
- Carbohydrates: 30g
- Fat: 10g
- Sodium: 450mg
- Potassium: 600mg
- Phosphorus: 220mg
- Portion Size: 1 serving

Roasted Vegetable Quiche

Ingredients:

- 1 pre-made whole wheat pie crust
- 1 cup cherry tomatoes, halved
- 1 cup zucchini, diced
- 1 cup bell peppers, diced
- 1/2 cup red onion, finely chopped
- 1 cup spinach, chopped
- 4 large eggs
- 1 cup low-fat milk
- 1 cup shredded Swiss cheese
- 1 teaspoon dried thyme

- Salt and pepper to taste

Instructions:

1. Preheat the oven to 375°F (190°C).

2. In a bowl, toss cherry tomatoes, zucchini, bell peppers, red onion, and spinach with olive oil, salt, and pepper.

3. Spread the vegetables on a baking sheet and roast for 20 minutes.

4. In a separate bowl, whisk together eggs, milk, shredded Swiss cheese, dried thyme, salt, and pepper.

5. Place the pre-made pie crust in a pie dish.

6. Arrange the roasted vegetables in the crust and pour the egg mixture over them.

7. Bake for 30-35 minutes or until the quiche is set and golden brown.

8. Allow it to cool slightly before slicing.

Nutrition Information:

- Calories: 320
- Protein: 15g

- Carbohydrates: 25g

- Fat: 18g

- Sodium: 450mg

- Potassium: 500mg

- Phosphorus: 200mg

- Portion Size: 1 slice

Chapter 4: Dinner Recipes

Welcome to Chapter 4 of the "Diabetic Renal Diet Cookbook," where we explore delightful dinner recipes designed to align with the principles of managing diabetes and renal health.

Baked Lemon Herb Chicken

Ingredients:

- 4 boneless, skinless chicken breasts
- 2 tablespoons olive oil
- 1 lemon, juiced
- 1 teaspoon dried thyme
- 1 teaspoon dried rosemary
- Salt and pepper to taste

Instructions:

1. Preheat the oven to 375°F (190°C).
2. In a bowl, mix olive oil, lemon juice, thyme, rosemary, salt, and pepper.

3. Place chicken breasts in a baking dish and coat with the herb mixture.

4. Bake for 25-30 minutes or until chicken is cooked through.

5. Serve with a side of steamed vegetables.

Nutrition Information:

- Calories: 250
- Protein: 30g
- Carbohydrates: 1g
- Fat: 13g
- Sodium: 120mg
- Potassium: 300mg
- Phosphorus: 150mg
- Portion Size: 1 chicken breast

Cauliflower Fried Rice with Shrimp

Ingredients:

- 1 cauliflower head, grated
- 1 cup shrimp, peeled and deveined
- 2 eggs, beaten
- 1 cup mixed vegetables (peas, carrots, corn)

- 2 tablespoons low-sodium soy sauce

- 1 tablespoon sesame oil

- 1 teaspoon ginger, minced

Instructions:

1. In a pan, cook shrimp until pink and set aside.

2. In the same pan, stir-fry cauliflower, mixed vegetables, and ginger.

3. Push vegetables to the side; scramble eggs on the other side.

4. Combine everything, add soy sauce and sesame oil, and stir well.

5. Mix in cooked shrimp and heat through.

Nutrition Information:

- Calories: 220

- Protein: 18g

- Carbohydrates: 10g

- Fat: 12g

- Sodium: 280mg

- Potassium: 400mg

- Phosphorus: 200mg

- Portion Size: 1 cup

Grilled Salmon with Dill Sauce

Ingredients:

- 4 salmon fillets
- 2 tablespoons olive oil
- 1 tablespoon fresh dill, chopped
- 1 clove garlic, minced
- Salt and pepper to taste

Instructions:

1. Preheat the grill to medium-high heat.
2. Rub salmon fillets with olive oil, garlic, dill, salt, and pepper.
3. Grill for 4-5 minutes per side or until salmon is flaky.
4. Serve with a dollop of dill sauce.

Nutrition Information:

- Calories: 300
- Protein: 25g
- Carbohydrates: 1g
- Fat: 20g

- Sodium: 100mg

- Potassium: 450mg

- Phosphorus: 250mg

- Portion Size: 1 salmon fillet

Vegetarian Zoodle Stir-Fry

Ingredients:

- 2 zucchinis, spiralized

- 1 cup tofu, cubed

- 1 bell pepper, thinly sliced

- 1 cup broccoli florets

- 2 tablespoons low-sodium soy sauce

- 1 tablespoon sesame oil

- 1 teaspoon ginger, grated

Instructions:

1. In a wok or skillet, sauté tofu until golden brown.

2. Add vegetables and ginger; stir-fry until tender-crisp.

3. Toss in zucchini noodles, soy sauce, and sesame oil.

4. Cook for an additional 2-3 minutes.

5. Garnish with sesame seeds and serve.

Nutrition Information:

- Calories: 180
- Protein: 12g
- Carbohydrates: 10g
- Fat: 10g
- Sodium: 300mg
- Potassium: 350mg
- Phosphorus: 150mg
- Portion Size: 1.5 cups

Stuffed Bell Peppers with Ground Turkey

Ingredients:

- 4 large bell peppers, halved
- 1 pound ground turkey
- 1 cup quinoa, cooked
- 1 cup black beans, drained and rinsed
- 1 cup diced tomatoes
- 1 teaspoon cumin
- 1 teaspoon chili powder
- Salt and pepper to taste

Instructions:

1. Preheat the oven to 375°F (190°C).

2. In a skillet, cook ground turkey until browned.

3. Mix in cooked quinoa, black beans, diced tomatoes, cumin, chili powder, salt, and pepper.

4. Stuff bell pepper halves with the turkey mixture.

5. Bake for 25-30 minutes or until peppers are tender.

Nutrition Information:

- Calories: 320
- Protein: 25g
- Carbohydrates: 30g
- Fat: 10g
- Sodium: 180mg
- Potassium: 550mg
- Phosphorus: 200mg
- Portion Size: 2 stuffed pepper halves

Roasted Garlic and Rosemary Pork Tenderloin

Ingredients:

- 1 pork tenderloin
- 3 cloves garlic, minced
- 2 tablespoons fresh rosemary, chopped
- 1 tablespoon olive oil
- Salt and pepper to taste

Instructions:

1. Preheat the oven to 400°F (200°C).
2. Make small incisions in the pork; insert minced garlic and rosemary.
3. Rub the pork with olive oil, salt, and pepper.
4. Roast for 25-30 minutes or until internal temperature reaches 145°F (63°C).
5. Let it rest before slicing.

Nutrition Information:

- Calories: 280
- Protein: 30g
- Carbohydrates: 1g
- Fat: 16g
- Sodium: 120mg
- Potassium: 400mg

- Phosphorus: 250mg
- Portion Size: 3 ounces

Eggplant Parmesan with Whole Wheat Pasta

Ingredients:

- 1 large eggplant, sliced
- 2 cups whole wheat pasta, cooked
- 1 cup marinara sauce (low sodium)
- 1 cup part-skim mozzarella, shredded
- 1/2 cup Parmesan cheese, grated
- 1 teaspoon dried oregano
- Fresh basil for garnish

Instructions:

1. Preheat the oven to 375°F (190°C).
2. Bake eggplant slices for 15 minutes, turning halfway.
3. In a baking dish, layer eggplant, cooked pasta, marinara sauce, and cheeses.
4. Repeat layers, finishing with a cheese layer on top.

5. Sprinkle with dried oregano and bake for 25-30 minutes.

Nutrition Information:

- Calories: 350
- Protein: 20g
- Carbohydrates: 40g
- Fat: 14g
- Sodium: 300mg
- Potassium: 500mg
- Phosphorus: 200mg
- Portion Size: 1.5 cups

Cilantro Lime Grilled Chicken

Ingredients:

- 4 boneless, skinless chicken breasts
- 1/4 cup fresh cilantro, chopped
- Zest and juice of 2 limes
- 2 tablespoons olive oil
- 1 teaspoon cumin
- Salt and pepper to taste

Instructions:

1. In a bowl, mix cilantro, lime zest, lime juice, olive oil, cumin, salt, and pepper.
2. Marinate chicken in the mixture for at least 30 minutes.
3. Preheat the grill to medium-high heat.
4. Grill chicken for 6-7 minutes per side or until fully cooked.
5. Serve with lime wedges.

Nutrition Information:

- Calories: 280
- Protein: 30g
- Carbohydrates: 2g
- Fat: 15g
- Sodium: 120mg
- Potassium: 400mg
- Phosphorus: 250mg
- Portion Size: 1 chicken breast

Quinoa and Vegetable Stuffed Peppers

Ingredients:

- 4 large bell peppers, halved
- 1 cup quinoa, cooked
- 1 cup black beans, drained and rinsed
- 1 cup cherry tomatoes, diced
- 1/2 cup corn kernels
- 1 teaspoon cumin
- 1 teaspoon smoked paprika
- Salt and pepper to taste

Instructions:

1. Preheat the oven to 375°F (190°C).
2. In a bowl, mix cooked quinoa, black beans, tomatoes, corn, cumin, smoked paprika, salt, and pepper.
3. Stuff bell pepper halves with the quinoa mixture.
4. Bake for 25-30 minutes or until peppers are tender.

Nutrition Information:

- Calories: 300
- Protein: 15g

- Carbohydrates: 55g

- Fat: 5g

- Sodium: 220mg

- Potassium: 500mg

- Phosphorus: 200mg

- Portion Size: 2 stuffed pepper halves

Blackened Tilapia with Mango Salsa

Ingredients:

- 4 tilapia fillets

- 2 teaspoons blackening seasoning

- 1 tablespoon olive oil

- 1 mango, diced

- 1/2 red onion, finely chopped

- 1 jalapeño, seeded and minced

- 2 tablespoons fresh cilantro, chopped

Instructions:

1. Rub tilapia fillets with blackening seasoning.

2. Heat olive oil in a skillet; cook tilapia for 3-4 minutes per side.

3. In a bowl, mix mango, red onion, jalapeño, and cilantro for salsa.

4. Top tilapia with mango salsa before serving.

Nutrition Information:

- Calories: 240
- Protein: 25g
- Carbohydrates: 15g
- Fat: 8g
- Sodium: 220mg
- Potassium: 400mg
- Phosphorus: 200mg
- Portion Size: 1 tilapia fillet

Spaghetti Squash with Tomato Basil Sauce

Ingredients:

- 1 large spaghetti squash
- 2 cups cherry tomatoes, halved
- 3 cloves garlic, minced
- 1/4 cup fresh basil, chopped

- 2 tablespoons olive oil

- Salt and pepper to taste

Instructions:

1. Preheat the oven to 375°F (190°C).

2. Cut the spaghetti squash in half lengthwise, scoop out seeds.

3. Place squash halves on a baking sheet, cut side down, and bake for 30-40 minutes.

4. In a skillet, sauté garlic in olive oil, add cherry tomatoes, and cook until soft.

5. Use a fork to scrape the spaghetti squash into strands; toss with tomato basil sauce.

Nutrition Information:

- Calories: 180

- Protein: 3g

- Carbohydrates: 30g

- Fat: 7g

- Sodium: 120mg

- Potassium: 350mg

- Phosphorus: 100mg

- Portion Size: 1 cup

Chicken and Vegetable Skewers

Ingredients:

- 1 pound chicken breast, cubed
- 1 zucchini, sliced
- 1 bell pepper, cut into chunks
- 1 red onion, cut into wedges
- 2 tablespoons olive oil
- 1 teaspoon smoked paprika
- 1 teaspoon dried oregano
- Salt and pepper to taste

Instructions:

1. Preheat the grill to medium-high heat.
2. In a bowl, mix chicken, zucchini, bell pepper, red onion, olive oil, smoked paprika, oregano, salt, and pepper.
3. Thread onto skewers and grill for 10-12 minutes, turning occasionally.
4. Serve with a side of quinoa or brown rice.

Nutrition Information:

- Calories: 280
- Protein: 25g
- Carbohydrates: 10g
- Fat: 15g
- Sodium: 180mg
- Potassium: 400mg
- Phosphorus: 200mg
- Portion Size: 2 skewers

Creamy Mushroom and Spinach Risotto

Ingredients:

- 1 cup Arborio rice
- 1/2 cup dry white wine
- 4 cups low-sodium vegetable broth, heated
- 1 cup mushrooms, sliced
- 2 cups fresh spinach, chopped
- 1/2 cup Parmesan cheese, grated
- 1 tablespoon olive oil
- 2 cloves garlic, minced

Instructions:

1. In a pan, sauté garlic in olive oil until fragrant.
2. Add Arborio rice and cook for 1-2 minutes.
3. Pour in white wine; stir until mostly absorbed.
4. Gradually add warm vegetable broth, stirring constantly until rice is cooked.
5. Stir in mushrooms, spinach, and Parmesan cheese until creamy.

Nutrition Information:

- Calories: 320
- Protein: 12g
- Carbohydrates: 45g
- Fat: 8g
- Sodium: 350mg
- Potassium: 300mg
- Phosphorus: 150mg
- Portion Size: 1 cup

Baked Cod with Lemon and Herbs

Ingredients:

- 4 cod fillets

- 2 tablespoons olive oil

- 1 lemon, sliced

- 2 teaspoons fresh thyme, chopped

- 1 teaspoon fresh dill, chopped

- Salt and pepper to taste

Instructions:

1. Preheat the oven to 400°F (200°C).

2. Place cod fillets in a baking dish; drizzle with olive oil.

3. Season with thyme, dill, salt, and pepper.

4. Arrange lemon slices on top of the fillets.

5. Bake for 15-20 minutes or until fish flakes easily.

Nutrition Information:

- Calories: 250

- Protein: 30g

- Carbohydrates: 1g

- Fat: 13g

- Sodium: 120mg

- Potassium: 400mg

- Phosphorus: 250mg

- Portion Size: 1 cod fillet

Teriyaki Tofu Stir-Fry

Ingredients:

- 1 block extra-firm tofu, pressed and cubed
- 2 cups broccoli florets
- 1 bell pepper, sliced
- 1 carrot, julienned
- 1/4 cup low-sodium teriyaki sauce
- 2 tablespoons soy sauce (low sodium)
- 1 tablespoon sesame oil
- 1 tablespoon ginger, minced

Instructions:

1. In a wok or skillet, stir-fry tofu until golden brown; set aside.
2. In the same pan, sauté ginger, broccoli, bell pepper, and carrot.
3. Add tofu back to the pan; pour in teriyaki sauce and soy sauce.
4. Stir-fry until vegetables are tender-crisp.
5. Drizzle with sesame oil before serving.

Nutrition Information:

- Calories: 280
- Protein: 15g
- Carbohydrates: 25g
- Fat: 14g
- Sodium: 400mg
- Potassium: 450mg
- Phosphorus: 200mg
- Portion Size: 1.5 cups

Chapter 5: Snacks and Appetizers

Welcome to Chapter 5 of the "Diabetic Renal Diet Cookbook," where we explore a delightful array of snacks and appetizers designed to tantalize your taste buds while adhering to the principles of a diabetic renal diet.

Guacamole with Veggie Sticks

Ingredients:

- 2 ripe avocados
- 1 small onion, finely diced
- 1 tomato, diced
- 1 clove garlic, minced
- 1 lime, juiced
- Salt and pepper to taste
- Assorted veggie sticks for dipping

Instructions:

1. Mash the avocados in a bowl.
2. Add diced onion, tomato, minced garlic, and lime juice.

3. Mix until well combined. Season with salt and pepper.

4. Serve with an assortment of veggie sticks.

Nutrition Information:

- Calories: 120
- Protein: 2g
- Carbohydrates: 8g
- Fat: 10g
- Sodium: 5mg
- Potassium: 350mg
- Phosphorus: 45mg
- Portion Size: 1/2 cup guacamole with veggie sticks.

Greek Yogurt and Cucumber Dip

Ingredients:

- 1 cup Greek yogurt
- 1 cucumber, finely diced
- 2 tablespoons fresh dill, chopped
- 1 clove garlic, minced
- Salt and pepper to taste

Instructions:

1. Mix Greek yogurt, diced cucumber, chopped dill, and minced garlic.

2. Season with salt and pepper.

3. Refrigerate for at least 30 minutes before serving.

Nutrition Information:

- Calories: 80
- Protein: 10g
- Carbohydrates: 6g
- Fat: 2g
- Sodium: 30mg
- Potassium: 200mg
- Phosphorus: 60mg
- Portion Size: 1/4 cup dip.

Hummus with Carrot and Celery Sticks

Ingredients:

- 1 can (15 oz) chickpeas, drained
- 3 tablespoons tahini

- 2 tablespoons olive oil

- 1 clove garlic, minced

- 1 teaspoon cumin

- Salt and lemon juice to taste

- Carrot and celery sticks for dipping

Instructions:

1. Blend chickpeas, tahini, olive oil, minced garlic, cumin, salt, and lemon juice until smooth.

2. Adjust seasoning to taste.

3. Serve with carrot and celery sticks.

Nutrition Information:

- Calories: 100

- Protein: 4g

- Carbohydrates: 10g

- Fat: 6g

- Sodium: 80mg

- Potassium: 120mg

- Phosphorus: 70mg

- Portion Size: 1/4 cup hummus with carrot and celery sticks.

Deviled Eggs with Avocado

Ingredients:

- 6 hard-boiled eggs, halved
- 1 ripe avocado
- 1 tablespoon Greek yogurt
- 1 teaspoon Dijon mustard
- Paprika for garnish

Instructions:

1. Remove egg yolks and mash with avocado, Greek yogurt, and mustard.
2. Spoon the mixture back into the egg whites.
3. Sprinkle with paprika for garnish.

Nutrition Information:

- Calories: 90
- Protein: 6g
- Carbohydrates: 4g
- Fat: 6g
- Sodium: 80mg
- Potassium: 220mg
- Phosphorus: 100mg

- Portion Size: 2 deviled egg halves.

Spicy Edamame

Ingredients:

- 2 cups edamame, steamed
- 1 tablespoon olive oil
- 1 teaspoon chili powder
- 1/2 teaspoon cayenne pepper
- Salt to taste

Instructions:

1. In a bowl, toss steamed edamame with olive oil, chili powder, cayenne pepper, and salt.
2. Ensure even coating and serve at room temperature.

Nutrition Information:

- Calories: 120
- Protein: 9g
- Carbohydrates: 8g
- Fat: 7g
- Sodium: 5mg
- Potassium: 250mg

- Phosphorus: 90mg

- Portion Size: 1 cup spicy edamame.

Cottage Cheese and Pineapple Skewers

Ingredients:

- 1 cup low-fat cottage cheese

- 1 cup fresh pineapple chunks

- Wooden skewers

Instructions:

1. Thread cottage cheese and pineapple alternately onto skewers.

2. Refrigerate for 20 minutes before serving.

Nutrition Information:

- Calories: 150

- Protein: 12g

- Carbohydrates: 15g

- Fat: 4g

- Sodium: 120mg

- Potassium: 180mg

- Phosphorus: 100mg

- Portion Size: 2 skewers.

Roasted Red Pepper and Feta Dip

Ingredients:

- 2 roasted red peppers, peeled and diced

- 1/2 cup feta cheese, crumbled

- 2 tablespoons Greek yogurt

- 1 clove garlic, minced

- 1 tablespoon olive oil

- Salt and pepper to taste

- Whole-grain pita chips for dipping

Instructions:

1. Combine roasted red peppers, feta, Greek yogurt, minced garlic, olive oil, salt, and pepper in a food processor.

2. Blend until smooth and creamy.

3. Serve with whole-grain pita chips.

Nutrition Information:

- Calories: 90
- Protein: 4g
- Carbohydrates: 6g
- Fat: 6g
- Sodium: 120mg
- Potassium: 100mg
- Phosphorus: 80mg
- Portion Size: 2 tablespoons dip with pita chips.

Almond and Pumpkin Seed Trail Mix

Ingredients:

- 1/2 cup almonds
- 1/2 cup pumpkin seeds
- 1/4 cup dried cranberries
- 1/4 cup dark chocolate chips
- 1/2 teaspoon cinnamon

Instructions:

1. Mix almonds, pumpkin seeds, dried cranberries, dark chocolate chips, and cinnamon in a bowl.
2. Store in an airtight container for a ready-to-go snack.

Nutrition Information:

- Calories: 160
- Protein: 5g
- Carbohydrates: 12g
- Fat: 10g
- Sodium: 5mg
- Potassium: 180mg
- Phosphorus: 70mg
- Portion Size: 1/4 cup trail mix.

Caprese Skewers with Balsamic Glaze

Ingredients:

- 1 cup cherry tomatoes
- 1 cup fresh mozzarella balls
- Fresh basil leaves
- Balsamic glaze for drizzling

Instructions:

1. Thread cherry tomatoes, fresh mozzarella balls, and basil leaves onto skewers.

2. Arrange on a serving platter and drizzle with balsamic glaze before serving.

Nutrition Information:

- Calories: 120
- Protein: 8g
- Carbohydrates: 6g
- Fat: 7g
- Sodium: 120mg
- Potassium: 180mg
- Phosphorus: 90mg
- Portion Size: 2 skewers.

Smoked Salmon Cucumber Bites

Ingredients:

- Cucumber slices
- Smoked salmon slices
- Cream cheese
- Fresh dill for garnish

Instructions:

1. Spread a thin layer of cream cheese on each cucumber slice.
2. Top with smoked salmon and garnish with fresh dill.

Nutrition Information:

- Calories: 90
- Protein: 6g
- Carbohydrates: 2g
- Fat: 7g
- Sodium: 180mg
- Potassium: 150mg
- Phosphorus: 70mg
- Portion Size: 3 pieces.

Kale Chips with Sea Salt

Ingredients:

- Fresh kale leaves, washed and dried
- Olive oil
- Sea salt

Instructions:

1. Preheat the oven to 350°F (175°C).
2. Remove stems from kale and tear leaves into bite-sized pieces.
3. Toss kale with olive oil and spread evenly on a baking sheet.
4. Sprinkle with sea salt.
5. Bake for 10-15 minutes or until the edges are crisp.

Nutrition Information:

- Calories: 50
- Protein: 3g
- Carbohydrates: 5g
- Fat: 3g
- Sodium: 200mg
- Potassium: 250mg
- Phosphorus: 40mg
- Portion Size: 1 cup.

Baked Sweet Potato Fries

Ingredients:

- 2 sweet potatoes, cut into fries

- 1 tablespoon olive oil

- 1 teaspoon paprika

- Salt and pepper to taste

Instructions:

1. Preheat the oven to 400°F (200°C).

2. Toss sweet potato fries with olive oil, paprika, salt, and pepper.

3. Spread evenly on a baking sheet and bake for 20-25 minutes or until golden.

Nutrition Information:

- Calories: 120

- Protein: 2g

- Carbohydrates: 25g

- Fat: 3g

- Sodium: 80mg

- Potassium: 350mg

- Phosphorus: 50mg

- Portion Size: 1 cup.

Avocado and Black Bean Salsa

Ingredients:

- 1 ripe avocado, diced
- 1 cup black beans, cooked and drained
- 1 cup corn kernels (fresh or frozen)
- 1/2 cup cherry tomatoes, halved
- 1/4 cup red onion, finely chopped
- Fresh cilantro, chopped
- Lime juice, to taste
- Salt and pepper, to taste

Instructions:

1. In a bowl, combine diced avocado, black beans, corn, cherry tomatoes, red onion, and cilantro.
2. Drizzle with lime juice and season with salt and pepper.
3. Gently toss until well mixed.

Nutrition Information:

- Calories: 130
- Protein: 5g
- Carbohydrates: 18g

- Fat: 5g

- Sodium: 200mg

- Potassium: 320mg

- Phosphorus: 80mg

- Portion Size: 1/2 cup.

Zucchini and Parmesan Crisps

Ingredients:

- 2 zucchinis, thinly sliced

- Grated Parmesan cheese

- Olive oil spray

- Garlic powder, to taste

- Dried oregano, to taste

Instructions:

1. Preheat the oven to 400°F (200°C).

2. Place zucchini slices on a baking sheet.

3. Sprinkle with Parmesan, garlic powder, and oregano.

4. Lightly spray with olive oil.

5. Bake for 15-20 minutes or until golden and crisp.

Nutrition Information:

- Calories: 70
- Protein: 4g
- Carbohydrates: 6g
- Fat: 4g
- Sodium: 120mg
- Potassium: 320mg
- Phosphorus: 60mg
- Portion Size: 1 cup.

Mixed Berry Smoothie Bowl

Ingredients:

- 1 cup mixed berries (strawberries, blueberries, raspberries)
- 1 banana, sliced and frozen
- 1/2 cup Greek yogurt
- 1/4 cup almond milk
- Toppings: granola, chia seeds, sliced almonds, fresh berries

Instructions:

1. In a blender, combine mixed berries, frozen banana, Greek yogurt, and almond milk.
2. Blend until smooth and creamy.
3. Pour into a bowl and top with granola, chia seeds, sliced almonds, and fresh berries.

Nutrition Information:

- Calories: 180
- Protein: 8g
- Carbohydrates: 30g
- Fat: 4g
- Sodium: 40mg
- Potassium: 380mg
- Phosphorus: 80mg
- Portion Size: 1 smoothie bowl.

Welcome to the delectable world of desserts crafted for the diabetic renal diet. Indulge your sweet cravings guilt-free with these carefully curated recipes that not only satisfy your taste buds but also align with the nutritional needs of managing diabetes and renal health.

Sugar-Free Berry Sorbet

Ingredients:

- 2 cups mixed berries (strawberries, blueberries, raspberries)
- 1/4 cup water
- 1 tablespoon lemon juice
- 1-2 tablespoons sugar substitute (as per taste)

Instructions:

1. Blend mixed berries, water, and lemon juice until smooth.
2. Add sugar substitute, adjusting sweetness to your preference.

3. Pour the mixture into a shallow dish and freeze for at least 4 hours.

4. Scoop and serve.

Nutrition Information (per serving):

- Calories: 70
- Protein: 1g
- Carbohydrates: 18g
- Fat: 0.5g
- Sodium: 2mg
- Potassium: 120mg
- Phosphorus: 20mg
- Portion Size: 1/2 cup

Dark Chocolate and Almond Clusters

Ingredients:

- 1/2 cup dark chocolate chips (sugar-free)
- 1/2 cup almonds, chopped

Instructions:

1. Melt dark chocolate chips in a heatproof bowl.

2. Stir in chopped almonds until well coated.

3. Spoon clusters onto a parchment-lined tray and refrigerate until set.

Nutrition Information (per serving):

- Calories: 120
- Protein: 3g
- Carbohydrates: 10g
- Fat: 8g
- Sodium: 5mg
- Potassium: 80mg
- Phosphorus: 50mg
- Portion Size: 2 clusters

Coconut and Chia Seed Pudding

Ingredients:

- 1/4 cup chia seeds
- 1 cup coconut milk (unsweetened)
- 1 teaspoon vanilla extract
- 1 tablespoon shredded coconut (unsweetened)

Instructions:

1. Mix chia seeds, coconut milk, and vanilla extract in a bowl.
2. Refrigerate for at least 2 hours or overnight.
3. Top with shredded coconut before serving.

Nutrition Information (per serving):

- Calories: 150
- Protein: 4g
- Carbohydrates: 10g
- Fat: 10g
- Sodium: 10mg
- Potassium: 90mg
- Phosphorus: 70mg
- Portion Size: 1/2 cup

Baked Apple with Cinnamon

Ingredients:

- 1 large apple, cored and sliced
- 1/2 teaspoon cinnamon
- 1 tablespoon chopped walnuts
- 1 tablespoon sugar substitute

Instructions:

1. Preheat the oven to 350°F (175°C).
2. Place apple slices in a baking dish and sprinkle with cinnamon.
3. Mix chopped walnuts with sugar substitute and sprinkle over the apples.
4. Bake for 20-25 minutes until apples are tender.

Nutrition Information (per serving):

- Calories: 80
- Protein: 1g
- Carbohydrates: 20g
- Fat: 1g
- Sodium: 0mg
- Potassium: 120mg
- Phosphorus: 15mg
- Portion Size: 1/2 apple

Greek Yogurt Cheesecake Bites

Ingredients:

- 1 cup Greek yogurt (unsweetened)
- 2 tablespoons cream cheese (reduced-fat)

- 1 tablespoon honey

- 1/2 teaspoon vanilla extract

Instructions:

1. In a bowl, mix Greek yogurt, cream cheese, honey, and vanilla extract until smooth.

2. Spoon the mixture into mini muffin cups and freeze until firm.

Nutrition Information (per serving):

- Calories: 60

- Protein: 3g

- Carbohydrates: 5g

- Fat: 3g

- Sodium: 30mg

- Potassium: 70mg

- Phosphorus: 40mg

- Portion Size: 2 bites

Avocado Chocolate Mousse

Ingredients:

- 1 ripe avocado

- 2 tablespoons unsweetened cocoa powder

- 3 tablespoons sugar substitute

- 1/2 teaspoon vanilla extract

Instructions:

1. Blend avocado, cocoa powder, sugar substitute, and vanilla extract until creamy.

2. Refrigerate for at least 2 hours before serving.

Nutrition Information (per serving):

- Calories: 100

- Protein: 2g

- Carbohydrates: 10g

- Fat: 7g

- Sodium: 5mg

- Potassium: 220mg

- Phosphorus: 40mg

- Portion Size: 1/2 cup

Pumpkin Pie Chia Pudding

Ingredients:

- 1/4 cup chia seeds

- 1 cup pumpkin puree
- 1 teaspoon pumpkin pie spice
- 2 tablespoons maple syrup (sugar-free)

Instructions:

1. Combine chia seeds, pumpkin puree, pumpkin pie spice, and maple syrup in a bowl.
2. Refrigerate for at least 2 hours or overnight.
3. Stir well before serving.

Nutrition Information (per serving):

- Calories: 90
- Protein: 3g
- Carbohydrates: 15g
- Fat: 3g
- Sodium: 5mg
- Potassium: 120mg
- Phosphorus: 70mg
- Portion Size: 1/2 cup

Berry and Almond Tart

Ingredients:

- 1 cup almond flour
- 2 tablespoons coconut oil (melted)
- 1 tablespoon sugar substitute
- 1 cup mixed berries (strawberries, blueberries, raspberries)

Instructions:

1. Mix almond flour, melted coconut oil, and sugar substitute to form a dough.
2. Press the dough into a tart pan and bake at 350°F (175°C) for 10 minutes.
3. Allow the crust to cool, then fill it with mixed berries.

Nutrition Information (per serving):

- Calories: 120
- Protein: 3g
- Carbohydrates: 8g
- Fat: 9g
- Sodium: 5mg
- Potassium: 80mg
- Phosphorus: 60mg
- Portion Size: 1/8 tart

Lemon Blueberry Parfait

Ingredients:

- 1 cup blueberries
- 1 cup Greek yogurt (unsweetened)
- Zest and juice of 1 lemon
- 1 tablespoon honey (optional)

Instructions:

1. In a glass, layer blueberries, Greek yogurt, lemon zest, and lemon juice.
2. Repeat the layers and drizzle with honey if desired.

Nutrition Information (per serving):

- Calories: 100
- Protein: 5g
- Carbohydrates: 15g
- Fat: 2g
- Sodium: 20mg
- Potassium: 150mg
- Phosphorus: 70mg
- Portion Size: 1 cup

Pistachio and Cranberry Energy Bites

Ingredients:

- 1/2 cup pistachios, finely chopped
- 1/2 cup dried cranberries (unsweetened)
- 1/4 cup almond butter
- 1 tablespoon chia seeds

Instructions:

1. Mix chopped pistachios, dried cranberries, almond butter, and chia seeds in a bowl.
2. Form into small bites and refrigerate for at least 1 hour.

Nutrition Information (per serving):

- Calories: 80
- Protein: 2g
- Carbohydrates: 8g
- Fat: 5g
- Sodium: 0mg
- Potassium: 60mg
- Phosphorus: 40mg

- Portion Size: 2 bites

Cinnamon Baked Pears

Ingredients:

- 2 ripe pears, halved and cored
- 1 teaspoon cinnamon
- 1 tablespoon chopped pecans
- 1 tablespoon honey (optional)

Instructions:

1. Preheat the oven to 375°F (190°C).
2. Place pear halves on a baking sheet, sprinkle with cinnamon, and top with chopped pecans.
3. Bake for 20-25 minutes until pears are tender.

Nutrition Information (per serving):

- Calories: 90
- Protein: 1g
- Carbohydrates: 20g
- Fat: 2g
- Sodium: 0mg
- Potassium: 120mg

- Phosphorus: 15mg
- Portion Size: 1/2 pear

Almond Flour Banana Bread

Ingredients:

- 1 cup almond flour
- 2 ripe bananas, mashed
- 2 eggs
- 1 teaspoon baking powder
- 1/2 teaspoon cinnamon

Instructions:

1. Mix almond flour, mashed bananas, eggs, baking powder, and cinnamon.
2. Pour the batter into a greased loaf pan and bake at 350°F (175°C) for 25-30 minutes.

Nutrition Information (per serving):

- Calories: 120
- Protein: 4g
- Carbohydrates: 10g
- Fat: 8g

- Sodium: 30mg

- Potassium: 130mg

- Phosphorus: 70mg

- Portion Size: 1 slice

Raspberry and Coconut Chia Jam

Ingredients:

- 1 cup raspberries

- 2 tablespoons chia seeds

- 1 tablespoon shredded coconut (unsweetened)

- 1-2 tablespoons honey (optional)

Instructions:

1. Mash raspberries and mix with chia seeds, shredded coconut, and honey.

2. Refrigerate for at least 1 hour before serving.

Nutrition Information (per serving):

- Calories: 70

- Protein: 2g

- Carbohydrates: 10g

- Fat: 3g

- Sodium: 0mg

- Potassium: 80mg

- Phosphorus: 40mg

- Portion Size: 2 tablespoons

Vanilla Bean Panna Cotta

Ingredients:

- 1 cup heavy cream

- 1/4 cup sugar substitute

- 1 vanilla bean, scraped

- 1 teaspoon gelatin

Instructions:

1. Heat heavy cream, sugar substitute, and vanilla bean in a saucepan until it simmers.

2. Remove from heat, add gelatin, and stir until dissolved.

3. Pour into molds and refrigerate for at least 4 hours.

Nutrition Information (per serving):

- Calories: 150

- Protein: 2g

- Carbohydrates: 2g
- Fat: 15g
- Sodium: 20mg
- Potassium: 60mg
- Phosphorus: 30mg
- Portion Size: 1/2 cup

Mint Chocolate Avocado Popsicles

Ingredients:

- 1 ripe avocado
- 1/4 cup cocoa powder (unsweetened)
- 1/4 cup mint leaves
- 1/4 cup almond milk (unsweetened)

Instructions:

1. Blend avocado, cocoa powder, mint leaves, and almond milk until smooth.
2. Pour into popsicle molds and freeze for at least 4 hours.

Nutrition Information (per serving):

- Calories: 80

- Protein: 2g

- Carbohydrates: 8g

- Fat: 6g

- Sodium: 5mg

- Potassium: 180mg

- Phosphorus: 40mg

- Portion Size: 1 popsicle

Chapter 7: Smoothies

These nutrient-packed smoothies offer a burst of flavors, blending health and deliciousness seamlessly. Each recipe is crafted with care, ensuring that the ingredients contribute to your well-being while satisfying your craving for a refreshing beverage.

Berry Blast Green Smoothie

Ingredients:

- 1 cup fresh mixed berries (strawberries, blueberries, raspberries)
- 1 cup spinach leaves, washed
- 1/2 banana
- 1/2 cup unsweetened almond milk
- Ice cubes

Instructions:

1. Combine berries, spinach, banana, and almond milk in a blender.
2. Blend until smooth.

3. Add ice cubes and blend again until desired consistency.

4. Pour into a glass and enjoy!

Nutrition Information (per serving):

- Calories: 120

- Protein: 4g

- Carbohydrates: 25g

- Fat: 2g

- Sodium: 50mg

- Potassium: 350mg

- Phosphorus: 80mg

- Portion Size: 1 smoothie

Tropical Turmeric Smoothie

Ingredients:

- 1 cup pineapple chunks

- 1/2 banana

- 1/2 teaspoon turmeric powder

- 1 tablespoon chia seeds

- 1 cup coconut water

- Ice cubes

Instructions:

1. Blend pineapple, banana, turmeric powder, chia seeds, and coconut water until smooth.
2. Add ice cubes and blend again until well combined.
3. Pour into a glass, and savor the tropical goodness!

Nutrition Information (per serving):

- Calories: 140
- Protein: 3g
- Carbohydrates: 30g
- Fat: 2.5g
- Sodium: 40mg
- Potassium: 300mg
- Phosphorus: 70mg
- Portion Size: 1 smoothie

Spinach and Pineapple Smoothie

Ingredients:

- 1 cup fresh pineapple chunks
- 1 cup fresh spinach leaves, washed
- 1/2 cup Greek yogurt (unsweetened)
- 1/2 teaspoon honey (optional)

- 1/2 cup water
- Ice cubes

Instructions:

1. Combine pineapple, spinach, Greek yogurt, honey (if using), and water in a blender.
2. Blend until smooth and creamy.
3. Add ice cubes and blend again for a refreshing texture.
4. Pour into a glass, and enjoy this green delight!

Nutrition Information (per serving):

- Calories: 110
- Protein: 5g
- Carbohydrates: 20g
- Fat: 2g
- Sodium: 30mg
- Potassium: 250mg
- Phosphorus: 60mg
- Portion Size: 1 smoothie

Blueberry Almond Butter Smoothie

Ingredients:

- 1 cup fresh blueberries
- 1 tablespoon almond butter
- 1/2 cup plain, unsweetened yogurt
- 1/2 cup almond milk
- 1 tablespoon flaxseeds
- Ice cubes

Instructions:

1. Blend blueberries, almond butter, yogurt, almond milk, and flaxseeds until smooth.
2. Add ice cubes and blend again for a creamy consistency.
3. Pour into a glass, and relish the delightful combination of blueberries and almond butter!

Nutrition Information (per serving):

- Calories: 150
- Protein: 6g
- Carbohydrates: 18g
- Fat: 7g

- Sodium: 40mg

- Potassium: 280mg

- Phosphorus: 75mg

- Portion Size: 1 smoothie

Cucumber and Mint Smoothie

Ingredients:

- 1 cup cucumber, peeled and chopped

- 1/4 cup fresh mint leaves

- 1/2 lime, juiced

- 1/2 cup plain Greek yogurt (unsweetened)

- 1/2 teaspoon agave syrup (optional)

- 1/2 cup water

- Ice cubes

Instructions:

1. Combine cucumber, mint leaves, lime juice, Greek yogurt, agave syrup (if using), and water in a blender.

2. Blend until smooth and refreshing.

3. Add ice cubes and blend again for a cool, crisp texture.

4. Pour into a glass, and enjoy the invigorating taste of cucumber and mint!

Nutrition Information (per serving):

- Calories: 90
- Protein: 5g
- Carbohydrates: 12g
- Fat: 2g
- Sodium: 25mg
- Potassium: 220mg
- Phosphorus: 50mg
- Portion Size: 1 smoothie

Chocolate Protein Smoothie

Ingredients:

- 1 scoop chocolate protein powder (low-sugar)
- 1 tablespoon almond butter
- 1/2 banana
- 1 cup unsweetened almond milk
- 1/2 teaspoon vanilla extract
- Ice cubes

Instructions:

1. Blend chocolate protein powder, almond butter, banana, almond milk, and vanilla extract until smooth and creamy.

2. Add ice cubes and blend again for a rich, chocolatey consistency.

3. Pour into a glass, and indulge in this protein-packed chocolate delight!

Nutrition Information (per serving):

- Calories: 180
- Protein: 15g
- Carbohydrates: 20g
- Fat: 7g
- Sodium: 60mg
- Potassium: 300mg
- Phosphorus: 120mg
- Portion Size: 1 smoothie

Mango and Ginger Smoothie

Ingredients:

- 1 cup fresh mango chunks

- 1 tablespoon fresh ginger, grated
- 1/2 cup plain, unsweetened yogurt
- 1/2 cup coconut water
- 1 tablespoon honey (optional)
- Ice cubes

Instructions:

1. Blend mango, grated ginger, yogurt, coconut water, and honey (if using) until smooth.
2. Add ice cubes and blend again for a tropical and invigorating texture.
3. Pour into a glass, and savor the exotic combination of mango and ginger!

Nutrition Information (per serving):

- Calories: 130
- Protein: 4g
- Carbohydrates: 28g
- Fat: 2g
- Sodium: 35mg
- Potassium: 280mg
- Phosphorus: 65mg

- Portion Size: 1 smoothie

Peach and Oatmeal Smoothie

Ingredients:

- 1 cup fresh peach slices
- 1/4 cup rolled oats (cooked and cooled)
- 1/2 cup plain Greek yogurt (unsweetened)
- 1/2 cup almond milk
- 1/2 teaspoon cinnamon
- Ice cubes

Instructions:

1. Blend peach slices, cooked oats, Greek yogurt, almond milk, and cinnamon until smooth.
2. Add ice cubes and blend again for a satisfying and wholesome texture.
3. Pour into a glass, and relish the comforting blend of peach and oatmeal!

Nutrition Information (per serving):

- Calories: 160
- Protein: 7g

- Carbohydrates: 25g

- Fat: 3g

- Sodium: 45mg

- Potassium: 290mg

- Phosphorus: 80mg

- Portion Size: 1 smoothie

Kiwi and Kale Smoothie

Ingredients:

- 2 kiwis, peeled and sliced

- 1 cup kale leaves, stems removed

- 1/2 green apple, cored and chopped

- 1/2 cup coconut water

- 1 tablespoon chia seeds

- Ice cubes

Instructions:

1. Combine kiwis, kale leaves, green apple, coconut water, and chia seeds in a blender.

2. Blend until smooth and vibrant.

3. Add ice cubes and blend again for a refreshing and nutrient-packed texture.

4. Pour into a glass, and enjoy the dynamic flavors of kiwi and kale!

Nutrition Information (per serving):

- Calories: 110
- Protein: 4g
- Carbohydrates: 22g
- Fat: 3g
- Sodium: 30mg
- Potassium: 260mg
- Phosphorus: 70mg
- Portion Size: 1 smoothie

Coconut and Berry Protein Smoothie

Ingredients:

- 1/2 cup mixed berries (strawberries, blueberries, raspberries)
- 1 scoop vanilla protein powder (low-sugar)
- 1/2 cup coconut milk (unsweetened)
- 1 tablespoon shredded coconut (unsweetened)
- 1/2 banana
- Ice cubes

Instructions:

1. Blend mixed berries, protein powder, coconut milk, shredded coconut, and banana until smooth.

2. Add ice cubes and blend again for a luscious and tropical texture.

3. Pour into a glass, and savor the combination of coconut and mixed berries!

Nutrition Information (per serving):

- Calories: 170
- Protein: 15g
- Carbohydrates: 20g
- Fat: 6g
- Sodium: 40mg
- Potassium: 280mg
- Phosphorus: 90mg
- Portion Size: 1 smoothie

Avocado and Spinach Smoothie

Ingredients:

- 1/2 ripe avocado
- 1 cup fresh spinach leaves, washed

- 1/2 cup plain Greek yogurt (unsweetened)
- 1/2 lime, juiced
- 1 tablespoon honey (optional)
- 1/2 cup water
- Ice cubes

Instructions:

1. Blend ripe avocado, spinach, Greek yogurt, lime juice, honey (if using), and water until smooth.
2. Add ice cubes and blend again for a creamy and nourishing texture.
3. Pour into a glass, and relish the velvety blend of avocado and spinach!

Nutrition Information (per serving):

- Calories: 140
- Protein: 5g
- Carbohydrates: 18g
- Fat: 7g
- Sodium: 30mg
- Potassium: 320mg
- Phosphorus: 70mg

- Portion Size: 1 smoothie

Watermelon and Mint Smoothie

Ingredients:

- 1 cup fresh watermelon cubes, seeds removed
- 1/4 cup fresh mint leaves
- 1/2 cup coconut water
- 1/2 cup plain, unsweetened yogurt
- 1 tablespoon chia seeds
- Ice cubes

Instructions:

1. Blend watermelon, mint leaves, coconut water, yogurt, and chia seeds until smooth.
2. Add ice cubes and blend again for a refreshing and hydrating texture.
3. Pour into a glass, and enjoy the cool and revitalizing taste of watermelon and mint!

Nutrition Information (per serving):

- Calories: 120
- Protein: 4g

- Carbohydrates: 22g

- Fat: 3g

- Sodium: 40mg

- Potassium: 280mg

- Phosphorus: 75mg

- Portion Size: 1 smoothie

Papaya and Lime Smoothie

Ingredients:

- 1 cup ripe papaya, peeled and cubed

- 1/2 lime, juiced

- 1/2 cup plain Greek yogurt (unsweetened)

- 1 tablespoon honey (optional)

- 1/2 cup coconut water

- Ice cubes

Instructions:

1. Blend ripe papaya, lime juice, Greek yogurt, honey (if using), and coconut water until smooth.

2. Add ice cubes and blend again for a tropical and invigorating texture.

3. Pour into a glass, and savor the delightful combination of papaya and lime!

Nutrition Information (per serving):

- Calories: 130
- Protein: 5g
- Carbohydrates: 25g
- Fat: 2g
- Sodium: 35mg
- Potassium: 300mg
- Phosphorus: 65mg
- Portion Size: 1 smoothie

Carrot Cake Smoothie

Ingredients:

- 1/2 cup carrots, peeled and chopped
- 1/2 banana
- 1/4 cup rolled oats
- 1/2 teaspoon cinnamon
- 1/2 cup almond milk
- 1 tablespoon walnuts, chopped
- Ice cubes

Instructions:

1. Blend carrots, banana, rolled oats, cinnamon, almond milk, and walnuts until smooth.

2. Add ice cubes and blend again for a hearty and satisfying texture.

3. Pour into a glass, and enjoy the reminiscent taste of carrot cake in a nutritious smoothie!

Nutrition Information (per serving):

- Calories: 160

- Protein: 5g

- Carbohydrates: 22g

- Fat: 7g

- Sodium: 40mg

- Potassium: 280mg

- Phosphorus: 80mg

- Portion Size: 1 smoothie

Coffee and Banana Protein Smoothie

Ingredients:

- 1/2 cup brewed coffee, cooled
- 1/2 banana
- 1 scoop vanilla protein powder (low-sugar)
- 1/2 cup almond milk
- 1 tablespoon almond butter
- Ice cubes

Instructions:

1. In a blender, combine brewed coffee, banana, vanilla protein powder, almond milk, and almond butter.
2. Blend until smooth and creamy.
3. Add ice cubes and blend again for a refreshing and energizing texture.
4. Pour into a glass, and enjoy the perfect fusion of coffee and banana with a protein boost!

Nutrition Information (per serving):

- Calories: 120
- Protein: 15g
- Carbohydrates: 10g
- Fat: 5g
- Sodium: 40mg

- Potassium: 240mg

- Phosphorus: 90mg

- Portion Size: 1 smoothie

CONCLUSION

As we reach the conclusion of the "Diabetic Renal Diet Cookbook," it's not just the end of a book but the beginning of a journey towards better health and well-being. This cookbook is not just a collection of recipes; it's a guide to transforming the way you approach food, ensuring that every meal is a celebration of health without compromising on taste.

In these pages, we've explored the intricacies of a diabetic renal diet, offering a diverse array of recipes that harmonize with the nutritional needs of those managing diabetes and renal health. From the vibrant breakfasts that kickstart your day to the comforting dinners that bring a sense of fulfillment, each dish has been carefully crafted to be delicious, nourishing, and supportive of your overall health goals.

The 30-day meal plan serves as a roadmap, providing structure and variety to make the transition to a healthier lifestyle seamless. As you navigate through the chapters, you'll discover the joy of creating meals that not only satisfy your taste buds but also contribute to your well-being.

Our snacks and appetizers section demonstrates that indulgence can be both guilt-free and delightful, showcasing inventive combinations that make snacking an enjoyable part of your day. Desserts take a sweet turn with treats that redefine what it means to have a satisfying post-meal experience, proving that sweetness can be enjoyed without compromising on health.

The smoothie section adds a refreshing touch, offering a rainbow of flavors that are not just nutritious but invigorating, providing a perfect blend of taste and vitality.

In closing, this cookbook is an invitation to savor every moment, every flavor, and every bite on your journey to health. It's a reminder that taking care of your body doesn't mean sacrificing the pleasure of eating; rather, it's an opportunity to explore a world of culinary possibilities that contribute to your overall well-being.

May this cookbook be a constant companion in your kitchen, inspiring you to experiment, innovate, and relish the path to a healthier, happier you. Here's to embracing health through the vibrant and flavorful tapestry of the "Diabetic Renal Diet Cookbook."